Healthy Hemp

Delicious Recipes for Using Hemp Foods

From the
WOODLAND EDITORS

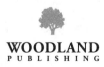

WOODLAND
PUBLISHING

For ordering information, contact:
Woodland Publishing
448 East 800 North, Orem, Utah 84097
www.woodlandpublishing.com

ISBN 1-58054-402-9
Printed in the United States of America

Contents

Hemp: An Introduction

Until recently, hemp was one of the most popular and highly valued crops in human society. For various reasons, it fell out of favor during the latter half of the twentieth century. Today, however, this very useful plant appears to be making a comeback.

The hemp plant is not only one of the oldest cultivated plants, it is also one of the most versatile and controversial plants known to man. Industrial hemp has a long history and has proven very valuable. Its stalks and seeds are being used as raw materials for a diverse array of products, including textiles and food. The plant's Latin name—*Cannabis sativa*—actually means "useful hemp," and it definitely lives up to its name!

What Is Hemp?

Cannabis sativa, is an annual belonging to the nettle family. It grows from five to fifteen feet in height with rich dark-green leaves composed of five to nine serrated, narrow, tapering leaflets that are pointed at the end and measure two to five inches in length and approximately one-third to one inch in width. When cultivated for industrial purposes, the plants are planted only inches apart: approximately nine hundred plants to the square yard. This results in the plants growing tall and having most of their leaves near the top.

Cannabis sativa will grow almost anywhere, requires little fertilizer, resists pests and crowds out weeds, therefore it is a crop that is relatively easy to grow and does well as an organic crop. The plant grows quickly, requiring only 70 to 110 days to mature. Due to this fact, industrial hemp is an abundant supplier of its extremely valuable raw materials, and is considered an important crop in the sustainable agricultural movement.

What Are the Differences Between Industrial Hemp and Marijuana?

Industrial hemp should not be confused with its "cousin" marijuana. Though they are essentially the same plant, there are substantial differences in how industrial hemp and marijuana are cultivated, thereby resulting in important differences in their end products. As mentioned earlier, the industrial hemp plant is usually planted very close together, which results in a taller, slender plant with branches at the top. This allows for a high yield of fiber in the stalk, which can be used for various commercial purposes, including clothing, paper and packaging products, furniture and other textiles. In contrast to the industrial hemp plant, the marijuana plant is usually planted yards apart, thereby resulting in it being quite dense, leafier, shorter, and bushier.

In addition, the close planting pattern results in a very low content of the compound THC (tetrahydrocannabinol), which is responsible for the psychoactive traits present in street-grade marijuana. Because the plant must focus its energy on growing tall to receive adequate sunlight, little energy is used to produce THC. And finally, industrial hemp plants contain much higher amounts of the non-psychoactive compound cannabidiol (CBD), which actively blocks the psychoactive effects of THC. When hemp food products are tested by independent labs with sensitive equipment, no THC can be detected.

Hemp: A Nutrient-Rich Package

The nutritional content of the hemp seed is impressive, offering 30 percent complete and highly digestible protein and containing over 36 percent essential fatty acids (which is approximately 16 percent more than flaxseed). Hemp seed contains protein, lipids, choline, inositol, enzymes, vitamins, minerals, phospholipids, phytosterols, and all eight essential amino acids. In fact, its amino acid profile is superior to that of soybeans, human milk, and cow's milk.

The complete protein in the hemp seed not only provides all the essential amino acids required to maintain health, it is 65 percent globulin edestin, contains albumin, and it is remarkably similar to the protein found in human blood plasma. Hemp oil also contains the carotenes and vitamin E (mixed tocopherols) that are naturally present in the seed.

Some experts suggest that hemp seed is one of the most nutritionally complete foods available today. Hemp seed could provide all the protein, carbohydrates, and essential fatty acids you need. However, for a nutritionally complete meal, you would need to combine it with foods high in vitamins (such as green, leafy vegetables) and minerals (such as roots) and other various micronutrients.

The following table provides a nutrient breakdown of 100 grams of hemp seed.

Did You Know? Hemp Facts

- Hemp is among the oldest industries on the planet, going back more than 10,000 years. The Columbia History of the World states that the oldest relic of human industry is a bit of hemp fabric dating back to approximately 8,000 B.C.
- Presidents Washington and Jefferson both grew hemp. Americans were legally bound to grow hemp during the Colonial Era and Early Republic.
- The original drafts of the Declaration of Independence and the Constitution were written on hemp paper.
- Hemp was used to create money in the Americas until the early 1800s.
- Henry Ford used hemp to build parts and create fuel for a car.
- The federal government subsidized hemp production during World War II and American farmers grew about a million acres of hemp as part of that program.
- Hemp produces more pulp per acre than timber on a sustainable basis, and can be used for every quality of paper. Hemp's low lignin content reduces the need for acids used in pulping, and its creamy color lends itself to environmentally friendly bleaching instead of harsh chlorine compounds. Less bleaching results in less dioxin and fewer chemical byproducts (toxins).
- Hemp fiber paper does not yellow with age when an acid-free process is used. Hemp paper more than 1,500 years old has been found. It can also be recycled more times than normal paper.
- China is currently the largest exporter of hemp paper and textiles. The fabrics are of excellent quality.

- Hemp seed is similar nutritionally to the soybean, containing more essential fatty acids than any other source, and being second only to soybeans in complete protein. Hemp seed is high in B vitamins and is 35 percent dietary fiber. Hemp seed is not psychoactive and cannot be used as a drug.

Nutritional Analysis of 100 grams of Hemp Seed

Calories	567
Protein	33 g
Saturated Fat	5 g
Monounsaturated Fat	5 g
Polyunsaturated Fat	36 g
Carbohydrate	12 g
Cholesterol	0 g
Total Dietary Fiber	6 g
Total Sugars	2 g
Vitamin A (B-Carotene)	4 IU
Thiamine (Vit. B1)	1.4 mg
Riboflavin (Vit. B2)	0.3 mg
Vitamin B6	0.1 mg
Vitamin C	1 mg
Vitamin E (d-A-tocopherol)	9 IU
Sodium	9 mg
Calcium	74 mg
Iron	4.7 mg

Hemp and Essential Fatty Acids:
A Superior Source

Hemp oil contains superior nutritional and therapeutic components and is an extremely healthful addition to one's diet. Hemp seed oil is more than 75 percent essential fatty acids in a well-balanced 3:1 ratio of omega-6 to omega-3. Like the seeds, it also contains GLA (gamma-linolenic acid). In his book, *Fats that Heal, Fats that Kill*, Udo Erasmus states that "hemp seed oil can be used over the long term to maintain a healthy EFA balance without leading to either EFA deficiency or imbalance."

There are two essential fatty acids: alpha linolenic acid and linoleic acid. In hemp seed, the two are found in the same ratio that many nutritionists agree is ideal for the human body's EFA requirements.

Alpha linolenic acid is an omega-3 superunsaturated essential fatty acid. As vital and beneficial as it is for the body, it can be found in significant amounts only in such seeds as chia, black currant, flax and kukui. Canola and pumpkin seed oils contain smaller amounts. Hemp seed oil is composed of about 19 percent alpha linolenic acid, compared to canola at about 9 percent

The other essential fat, linoleic acid, is an omega-6 polyunsaturated fat that is more common in foods than alpha linolenic acid. Linoleic acid comprises about 57 percent of hemp seed oil. Besides these two essential fatty acids, hemp oil contains other fatty acids that are very helpful in maintaining optimal health. The following provides a complete breakdown of hemp oil's fatty acid profile:

Fatty Acid Profile for Hemp Oil

Omega-3 (Alpha-Linolenic)	19.0%
Omega-6 (Linoleic)	57.0%
Omega-9 (Oleic)	12.0%
Gamma-linolenic (GLA)	1.7%
Stearic Acid	2.0%
Palmitic	6.0%
Other	2.3%

According to many experts, hemp seed is the richest plant source of essential fatty acids and contains a relatively low percentage of saturated fats. The essential fats in the oil and seeds perform of variety of functions within the human body. These include aiding cellular growth, promoting healthy skin, hair, and eyes, and assisting in immune function, proper weight control, and cognitive functions. The human brain is 60 percent fat; therefore, many of the essential fats are critical to its proper function and good health. Essential fatty acids are also the raw material required by the body to produce hormones, the body's communication network for cellular activity.

Deficiencies in essential fatty acids can lead to a variety of health problems. They include (but aren't limited to) the following: impairment of vision and neurological function, growth retardation, rheumatoid arthritis, hypertension, sticky blood platelets, lack of motor coordination, tingling sensation in arms and legs, high triglycerides, tissue inflammation, edema, dry skin, atopic eczema and psoriasis, acne, hair loss, skin eruptions, ulcerative colitis and Crohn's disease, liver and/or kidney degeneration, osteoporosis, susceptibility to infections, sterility in males, miscarriage, premenstrual syndrome, hormone imbalance, and impaired wound healing and cell growth. Numerous studies exist demonstrating that many common conditions and illnesses are related to fatty acid deficiencies and that dietary supplementation of EFAs, particular-

Hemp: A Brief History

- The use of hemp can be traced back to 8,000 B.C. in the Middle East and China where the fiber was used for textiles, the oil for cosmetic purposes and the seeds for food. From as early as five years before Christ was born to the mid-1800s hemp fibers were used to manufacture a large majority (some say up to 90 percent) of all ships' canvas sails, rigging, nets, and caulk. Hemp was also used for making paper, twines, carpet thread, carpet yarns, sailcloth, and for homespun and similar grades of woven goods.

- The Pilgrims first brought hemp seeds to America in 1632 and by 1850 hemp was America's third largest crop. In fact, early American farmers were required to grow it.

- Hemp was formally christened *Cannabis sativa L.* in 1753 by Swedish botanist Carl Linnaeus.

- In 1916 the U.S. Department of Agriculture issued an urgent warning stating that the country did not have enough forest land to sustain its needs. The bulletin containing this warning, also offered a profitable solution: "Grow more hemp! Virtually anything made of wood can also be made with hemp and it has a much higher sustainable yield."

- As hemp cultivation flourished in many countries, Britain declared it illegal in 1928.

- The existence of industrial hemp's botanical cousin, marijuana, which contains high levels of psychoactive substances, further impaired hemp's standing.

- In 1938 Canada followed suit and banned hemp farming. As most Western countries banned hemp, hemp farming and production continued in Eastern Europe, China, and a few other Asian countries.

- During World War II, the Canadian and American governments briefly lifted the restrictions on hemp farming to aid the war effort and boost the economy. At the end of the war, hemp farming was again banished.
- In 1993 Britain legalized hemp farming once again and in 1994 Health Canada issued the first research permit for growing industrial hemp. In 1998 hemp farming was again legalized in Canada. This has already helped many of Canada's farmers save their farms and added a valuable resource back into Canada's economy.
- To date hemp cultivation continues its illegal status in the United States. Recently there has been an encouraging development: California, Colorado, Hawaii, Kansas, North Dakota and Missouri have introduced or passed legislation to legalize the cultivation of industrial hemp in their states.

ly if included with a healthful, whole foods diet, will often prevent, improve, or cure these illnesses.

Supplementation of EFAs (including hemp oil) could also be a beneficial therapy for those suffering with cancer, diabetes, chronic depression, postpartum depression, attention deficit disorder and schizophrenic psychosis.

How Are Hemp Food Products Created?

With the recent emergence of hemp foods—mainly protein flour, oil and seed/nut products—one may wonder how these food products are produced. These nutritious foods are derived from the seed of the hemp plant, which as previously stated, are tested to ensure they are free of THC, the psychoactive substance present in "marijuana."

Technically speaking, the seed of the hemp plant is called an "achene," a fruit that is small and dry and usually contains an oily germ. The hard hull of an achene usually has no nutritional value and is often removed before consumption. (One only has to imagine a baseball player spitting out the shells of sunflower seeds, another example of an achene.) Hemp seed hulls are relatively easy for humans to chew and digest; however, shelled or hulled hemp seed is increasingly becoming more popular and is emerging as a main form of hemp food.

Hemp Seed

Hemp seeds are tiny nuts within shells or hulls that develop in the female flower of the plant. When they mature, they develop a thin, crunchy hull. This hull protects the seed's embryo and is composed mainly of fiber and chlorophyll.

The nut or seed represents the seed's center for storage of energy and building materials. Proteins, amino acids, oil and carbohydrates comprise the bulk of the nutSmaller amounts of vitamins and minerals make up the rest of the nut.

Hemp seeds can be eaten whole. Usually they are toasted and eaten much like popcorn, or they can be cooked in with other foods. Hemp nuts are hemp seeds that have had the hulls removed. They are becoming quite popular as a nutritious snack, both for their "nutty" taste and for the convenience of not having the sometimes bothersome hull included. They can be used raw, toasted, baked or ground and substituted for just about any other seed or nut used in cooking. The emp nut's delicious flavor is usually described somewhere 'ween a walnut and a sesame seed.

'emp seeds (or nuts) have many delightful applications in ilinary field. They can be substituted for dairy, soy or rice protein in the production of nondairy beverages, frozen desserts, tofu, and cheeses. Toasting lightly enhances the delicious nutty flavor of the seeds, but eating them raw will preserve all the nutrients. Hemp seeds can be sprinkled on salads, vegetables, pasta, or added to smoothies, granola, baked goods, soups, sauces, dips, salad dressings, and nut balls. Another great use for the seeds is to make them into hemp nut butter (see sidebar on page 36).

Hemp Protein (Hemp Flour or Hemp Meal)

Hemp protein (also referred to as hemp flour, meal or protein powder) is the finely ground seed meal that remains when seeds are pressed for oil. It typically contains 5 to 10 percent oil, with the rest being protein and hulls. Since hemp protein is high in oil, lacks gluten and has a very pungent flavor, it is recommended to use hemp protein flour as an additive to other flours. These include unbleached white, whole wheat, oats, barley, millet, quinoa, amaranth, rice lentil, corn, chickpea, chestnut, or rye flours. Typically a ratio of one part hemp protein flour to two or three parts other flour is recommended. Because of its high oil content, rancidity can be a problem with hemp protein flour. Consequently, it is recommended to keep the flour cool, dry and tightly sealed (the refrigerator or freezer are great places to store it). Shelf life of hemp protein flour should be over a year if kept under these conditions.

Hemp flour/meal is high in various nutrients, especially protein, essential amino acids and EFAs (essential fatty acids). Because of this, many people use the protein flour much in the same way soy flour is used as a replacement for wheat flour. Hemp flour also contains vitamins A, E, C, D, B2, B6, B1, boron, manganese, iron, potassium, magnesium, calcium, and zinc. Another attractive aspect of hemp protein flour is

Hemp Foods: Can You Get "High"?

One of the questions often asked concerning hemp foods is whether they contain any psychoactive substances. New industrial plant varieties contain an extremely small percentage (0.1%) of THC (tetrahydrocannabinol) in the sticky resin produced by the flowering tops of the female plants before the seeds mature. However, the strains of hemp grown for commercial purposes have an extremely low resin content. And if the seeds are hulled and cleaned for use in various products (which is how the large majority of hemp seed foods are sold in today's market), there is virtually no THC remaining—certainly not enough to create any psychoactivity. Recent research confirms that people who eat hemp food are extremely unlike to test positive for THC in workplace testing.

that it's often considered a "raw" food since the whole seed and hull are crushed at low temperatures to protect the valuable oil, nutrients and living enzymes.

Hemp flour is extremely versatile when it comes to food. It can be used in virtually all baking that involves flour (though it is best used mixed with other grain flours). Hemp protein flour can be used in breads, muffins, cakes, gravies, sauces, desserts, and many other dishes to increase nutritional content.

Hemp Oil

Hemp oil is obtained from the hemp seed. The oil contains essential fatty acids to maintain healthy human life. acids are essential because the body can't produce them independently—thus, they must be obtained through one's diet. EFAs have various roles in the body. They provide the raw materials from which hormones are comprised. EFAs are also critical to the proper functioning of individual cells, and the lack of EFAs are linked to a variety of health conditions, including eczema, cardiovascular disease, rheumatoid arthritis, osteoporosis, psoriasis and many more. Some experts maintain that hemp seed oil contains the ideal ratio of essential fatty acids (3 to 1 of omega-6 to omega-3).

One caveat with hemp seed oil is that because of its high content of polyunsaturated fats, it is fairly unstable. Thus, extra care is required to ensure that is does not turn rancid. Heat, light and oxygen are natural enemies of the oil. Consequently, the oil should be stored in dark containers and kept in cool, dry places, such as the refrigerator. Shelf life should be at least eight months if these recommendations are heeded.

Hemp oil can be integrated into the diet in various healthy ways. Use in the preparation of salad dressings, marinades, dips, spreads, add to smoothies, drizzle on any food such as potatoes and cooked grains, or simply take by the spoonful as an important addition to a healthy diet. Hemp oil has a very pleasant, nutty taste similar to sunflower oil.

Clearly, hemp food products contain important nutrients that are vital to human health and well being. They not only taste great, but they are very nutritious and versatile in their applications. Hemp is truly an amazing plant!

HEMP RECIPES

The main purpose of these recipes is to highlight the versatility and health benefits of hemp. However, there are various ways to adapt the recipes to better fit one's own health perspective. The following list provides some more healthful alternatives for some of the ingredients that may be found in these recipes.

Ingredient	Alternative
yogurt	soy yogurt
dairy milk	soy, hemp seed, rice or nut milk
eggs	egg substitute or flax seeds
butter	non-hydrogenated margarine
sugar	raw, organic or turbinado sugar
honey	maple syrup, barley malt or brown rice syrup
all-purpose/white flour	whole wheat or unbleached flour
baking powder	non-aluminum baking powder

Basic Hemp Vinaigrette

2/3 cup hemp seed oil
1 tablespoon balsamic vinegar
1 tablespoon lime or lemon juice
1 tablespoon orange juice
1/8 teaspoon cumin
salt to taste

ix all ingredients in a glass jar or dressing bottle. Can store
used for about two weeks.

Blueberry Hemp Salad Dressing

1/2 cup blueberries
1/2 cup hemp seed oil
1/2 cup water
3 tablespoons hemp seeds
2 tablespoons apple cider vinegar

Blend all ingredients together and enjoy!

Hemp Banana Power Smoothie

1 banana
4 strawberries
1/2 mango
1/3 cup plain yogurt (or soy yogurt)
2 tablespoons hemp protein flour (or 1/8 cup hemp nuts)
1/3 cup crushed ice
1–2 tablespoons honey, agave nectar or maple syrup

Blend banana, mango, strawberries and yogurt together in a blender and blend until smooth. Add hemp flour, crushed ice and honey. Blend until smooth. Adjust ingredients to taste. Makes 32 oz.

Hemp-Blueberry Shake

1 cup frozen blueberries
1 cup hemp milk
1 cup crushed ice
1 tablespoon hemp seed oil
1/4 cup pure maple syrup (do not use artificially flavored "maple" syrups)
1 1/2 teaspoons natural vanilla extract
1 heaping tablespoon toasted hemp seed

Blend ingredients in blender until smooth. Adjust ingredients to taste. Honey or agave nectar may be substituted for the maple syrup.

Strawberry-Kiwi Hemp Smoothie

1 cup skim milk (soy or rice milk can be substituted)
1 ripe banana
2 tablespoons hemp protein powder
2 tablespoons fresh lemon juice
4 tablespoons honey
1/3 cup fresh or frozen strawberries
1 kiwi fruit, peeled
1 cup ice

Blend all ingredients until smooth. Serve immediately. Pure 'ple syrup or agave nectar may be substituted for the honey.

Orange Hemp Smoothie

1 cup ice
2 cups vanilla soy milk
2 tablespoons hemp protein powder
1/4 cup soft tofu
1 cup fresh orange juice
1/4 cup pure maple syrup
1 ripe banana
1/2 teaspoon cinnamon or nutmeg (optional)

Blend all ingredients except cinnamon/nutmeg on high until smooth. Sprinkle cinnamon/nutmeg on top, and serve immediately. Honey or agave nectar may be substituted for the maple syrup.

Hemp Custard

1 cup milk
1 cup hulled hemp seed
1/8 cup maple syrup
1 egg and 1 egg yolk

Pre-heat oven to 275°F.
Place milk in a small pot and bring to a boil then remove from heat.
Place hemp seed in a small bowl and pour the milk and maple syrup in with the hulled hemp seed, cover lightly with plastic wrap.
Let rest for 10 minutes, then place ingredients in a blender at high speed for 3 minutes or until smooth.
Remove ingredients from the blender and place in a small bowl. Add the eggs and beat with a whisk.

Place hemp mixture in four 4-ounce ramekins or coffee cups and place in an ovenproof pot with hot water halfway up the sides of the ramekins or coffee cups.

Cover pot and place in oven.

Bake for 30 to 35 minutes or until firm when you wiggle the custard.

Remove from the pot and refrigerate.

Serve when cool. Makes 3 servings.

Chi Hemp Industries Incorporated, www.chii.ca

Hemp Crepe Batter

1/2 cup all-purpose flour
1/2 cup hemp protein flour
1 teaspoon cornstarch
2 cups of milk
1/8 teaspoon salt
2 eggs
1 egg yolk
1/4 cup butter

Place all dry ingredients in a medium-sized bowl and mix thoroughly.

Add eggs and milk and whisk until smooth.

Melt butter in a small pot or saucepan, add to flour and add to liquid mixture and beat with a whisk until well incorporated. Place in fridge for 30 minutes.

Remove from fridge and beat with a whisk before using.

Place a medium non-stick pan on medium heat.

Add 2 ounces of crepe batter to non-stick pan.

Cook on one side for about 90 seconds and flip gently with a spatula.

Cook one more minute and place on a plate until ready to use. Makes 15 large crepes.

Chi Hemp Industries Incorporated, www.chii.ca

Toasted Apple Cinnamon Hemp Cereal

1 cup oats (uncooked)
1/2 cup hemp protein powder (hemp flour)
1/2 cup flax seeds, ground
1/2 cup sunflower seeds
1/2 cup sesame seeds
1/2 cup almonds, diced
1/2 apple, diced
1/2 cup hemp oil
1/2 cup molasses
2 teaspoons apple juice
1 1/2 teaspoons cinnamon
1/2 teaspoon nutmeg
1/2 teaspoon whole stevia leaf, dried and ground
1/2 teaspoon sea salt

Preheat oven to 250°F. Mix all dry ingredients together. Blend liquid ingredients until they reach a consistent texture. Combine liquid and dry ingredients. Mix well. Spread on a baking tray. Bake for 1 hour. Let cool, break up. Keep refrigerated to extend freshness.

(Note: You'll notice that this cereal is toasted at a lower temperature than traditional granola. The reason for this is to preserve the essential fatty acids. Heating foods with essential fatty acids above 350°F is not recommended since the heat can convert EFAs to trans fats.)

Apple Ginger Hemp Snacks

1/2 cup dates
1 tablespoon fresh ginger
1/2 small apple
3 tablespoons hemp seeds
2 tablespoons ground flax seeds
3 tablespoons sesame seeds for outside coating

Process everything in a food processor (except sesame seeds). Form into flat, bar-like pieces or roll into small bite size balls, and roll or press in sesame seeds.

Let sit out overnight to dry.

These are quick and easy to make, with no baking necessary. An excellent post-workout alternative to conventional energy bars, these snacks are much healthier.

www.brendanbrazier.com

Root Vegetable Hemp Cakes

1 large or 2 medium parsnips, peeled
1 medium carrot, peeled
3 shiitake mushrooms
1 small onion, peeled
1 cup hulled hemp seed
1/4 cup hemp protein flour
1 clove of garlic sliced thin
1 tablespoon minced ginger
2 green onions sliced in 1/4 inch pieces

Preheat oven to 300°F. Cut parsnip in half lengthwise. If it is a large parsnip, cut it into 4 pieces; cut carrot lengthwise in half.

Quarter onion. Place carrots, parsnips and onions on a well-oiled baking sheet and place in oven. After 10 minutes add shiitake mushrooms.

Bake for 10-15 more minutes or until everything is soft. Remove from oven and let cool to room temperature.

Place all ingredients in a food processor and puree for 3 minutes. Remove ingredients from processor, place in a medium sized bowl and refrigerate for 30 minutes. Form mixture into two 6-ounce patties or four 3-ounce patties.

Place medium frying pan on medium heat with 2 ounces of oil in it; flour each side of the patty and fry until golden brown on each side.

Place patty in a 350°F oven for 5 minutes and serve. Makes 3–4 patties.

Chi Hemp Industries Incorporated, www.chii.ca

Hemp Tortillas

2 cups all-purpose flour
2 cups hemp protein flour
6 tablespoons corn oil
1 teaspoon cornstarch
3/4 to 1 cup warm water
salt and pepper

Combine flours, salt, pepper and cornstarch, add corn oil and rub into flour with fingers until it resembles small peas. Add warm water a little at a time until the mixture forms a ball, not too wet or dry.

Let it rest at room temperature for 30 minutes.

Roll out thin and fry in a lightly oiled pan for 2 minutes each side. Makes 5 servings.

Chi Hemp Industries Incorporated, www.chii.ca

Hulled Hemp Seed Gomasio

2 cups hemp seed
6 teaspoons sea salt
cayenne pepper to taste

Lightly toast hemp seed in the oven. Mix in sea salt. Add a little cayenne pepper to taste. Makes a nice addition to any meal.

Chi Hemp Industries Incorporated, www.chii.ca

Power Hemp Popcorn

1 cup unpopped popcorn
hemp oil
nutritional yeast
balsamic vinegar
sea salt

Pop popcorn in an air popper.
To the bowl of popcorn add a liberal amount of hemp oil, nutritional yeast, balsamic vinegar (just a little), and sea salt to taste.

Chi Hemp Industries Incorporated, www.chii.ca

Banana Crumb Hemp Muffins

1/2 cup all-purpose flour
1 teaspoon baking soda
1 teaspoon baking powder
1/2 teaspoon salt
3 bananas, mashed
3/4 cup white sugar
1 egg, lightly beaten
1/3 cup butter, melted
1/3 cup packed brown sugar
1 tablespoon all-purpose flour
1/8 teaspoon ground cinnamon
1 tablespoon butter
1 cup hulled hemp seed

Preheat oven to 375°F. Lightly grease 10 muffin cups, or line with muffin papers.

In a large bowl, mix together flour, baking soda, baking powder and salt. In another bowl, beat together bananas, sugar, egg and melted butter. Stir the banana mixture into the flour mixture just until moistened. Spoon batter into prepared muffin cups.

In a small bowl, mix together brown sugar, flour, cinnamon and hulled hemp seed. Cut in butter until mixture resembles coarse cornmeal. Sprinkle topping over muffins.

Bake in preheated oven for 18 to 20 minutes, until a toothpick inserted into center of a muffin comes out clean. Makes 10 muffins.

Chi Hemp Industries Incorporated, www.chii.ca

Date Delights

medjool dates
hemp nut butter

Cut organic medjool dates in half lengthwise. Spread with 1 teaspoon hemp nut butter.

These simple and tasty morsels are perfect for potlucks or other gatherings!

tonyakay.com

Ants on a Log

organic celery
hemp nut butter
organic sun-dried raisins

Cut organic celery into 2-inch sticks. Fill each celery stick with hemp nut butter. Decorate with organic sun-dried raisins.

tonyakay.com

Deep Sea Shaker

1/2 cup hemp seeds
1/3 cup dulse flakes

Use this combination in place of salt. It's also great as a decorative topping on pates, pizza, cold salads, and soups.

tonyakay.com

Chocolate Chiquita

1 organic banana
raw carob powder
raw coconut flakes
hemp protein powder

Thickly slice banana. Generously coat with equal parts raw carob powder, raw coconut flakes, and hemp protein powder. Eat with chopsticks.
tonyakay.com

Hemp Guacamole

2 large ripe peeled avocados
2 medium tomatoes, diced
2 tablespoons lemon or lime juice
1/2 teaspoon chili powder
1/2 cup diced onion
1/4 cup hemp nuts
1 1/2 teaspoons fresh cilantro leaves, chopped finely
1/2 teaspoon salt

Mash the avocados with a fork and add lemon/lime juice. Finely chop the onion and tomatoes and add to the avocados. Add the salt, chili powder, hemp nuts and cilantro. Serve and enjoy!

Hemp Nut Burgers

1 cup hemp nuts
8–10 ounces soft tofu
1/4 cup white onion, chopped
1/4 cup sunflower seeds
2 tablespoons soy sauce
2 tablespoons nutritional yeast
2 cups bread stuffing
1 teaspoon basil, chopped (or 1/2 teaspoon dried)
1 teaspoon oregano, chopped (or 1/2 teaspoon dried)
1/2 teaspoon dried garlic

In a blender, puree tofu then add the rest of the ingredients except stuffing. In a bowl, place the stuffing tofu mixture. Mix well. Form into burger patties. Bake on a greased cookie sheet in a 300°F oven for 25 minutes or until golden brown. Or grill carefully until golden brown.

Wheat-Free Hemp Pancakes

2 cups hemp protein flour
1 cup corn flour
1 cup oat flour
1 cup brown rice flour
3 heaping tablespoons turbinado sugar
5 heaping teaspoons baking powder
1 teaspoon sea salt
6 tablespoons hemp seed oil
5 cups water
safflower oil

In a large bowl, combine all the ingredients (except the saf-flower oil) in order. Oil an iron skillet with safflower oil and heat it over a medium-high flame. Using a ladle or pitcher, drop the mixture onto the skillet into palm-sized round cakes. Peek under each cake. When golden brown in color, it's time to flip them. Cook only once on each side. Serve topped with fruit, yogurt, or favorite fruit syrup. Serves 6–8.

The Hemp Cookbook, Todd Dalotto

Seedy Sweeties

Seedy Sweeties were the main product my company, Hungry Bear Hemp Foods, produced and distributed throughout North America. Being the second hemp food product to come out on the market, this was the first taste of hemp seed for thousands of peo-ple. As they were loved and appreciated by many, I received countless requests for the recipe, which I politely declined. Now that they are no longer being produced, I can withhold the recipe no longer. Makes between two and three 11 x 17 cookie sheets.

1 1/3 cups sweet Barbados molasses
2/3 cup brown rice syrup
(or replace the above two syrups with 2 cups sorghum syrup if available)
2 cups whole or hulled hemp seed
2 cups oat flour
2 1/3 cups brown sesame seed
1 1/3 cups cashews (for nutty type), or sunflower seeds (for sunflower type)
1 cup Brazil nuts (for nutty type), or sunflower seeds (for sunflower type)
hemp seed oil

Oil your cookie sheets with hemp seed oil.

Combine the hemp seed, oat flour, 1 1/3 cups of the sesame seed, and the cashews (or sunflower seeds) in a wok or large, sturdy mixing bowl.

In a large saucepan, heat syrups at high heat. Insert candy thermometer so that the tip is submerged in the syrup, but not touching the pan. After a few minutes the syrups will begin to foam up. When this occurs, turn the heat down until the foam subsides, being careful not to get splattered. Return to high heat and partially cover. Check the temperature often. When the syrups reach 270°F (132°C) (the temperature can be varied from between 250°F [soft] to 300°F [hard] depending on your preferred hardness), remove from heat and immediately pour into the seed mix. Stir until consistent.

Quickly pour onto the oiled cookie sheets. Spread mixture as evenly as you can, then roll flat with a rolling pin oiled with hemp seed oil. If it gets sticky, just allow to cool for a few minutes, then try again. After fifteen minutes, cut into squares with a pizza cutter.

Combine the rest of the sesame seeds with the Brazil nuts (or sunflower seeds) and run the mixture through a steel hand-cranked food grinder with the medium-sized-hole plate. This will grind them into a coarse, oily meal.

When the treats are cool enough to work with, scrape each square from the cookie sheet, roll each in the ground seed, and serve. If you have difficulty removing treats from pans, warm the bottom of the pan.

The Hemp Cookbook, Todd Dalotto

Vegan Hemp Raspberry Cheese Cake

Paul Benhaim, formerly the managing director of New Earth Ltd., can often be found cruising neighborhoods and events in a hemp ice cream van serving sweet frozen hemp seed delights. This is a project of the Hemp Food Industries Association to promote hemp foods. Paul has also shared this great dessert recipe with us. Makes one 8-inch pie.

  2 cups crushed graham crackers, sweet granola or crushed
    crunchy cookies
  3/4 cup hemp protein flour
  1/2 stick (4 tablespoons) organic, non-hydrogenated margarine
  1 pound silken tofu
  3 tablespoons cane syrup or light honey
  1/2 cup raw cane sugar
  juice of 1 lemon
  pinch of sea salt
  2 teaspoons vanilla extract
  2 large bananas
  1/2 pound fresh raspberries

To make the crust, mix the crackers, hemp protein flour, and margarine in a food processor until they're combined. Pat the mixture into an 8-inch round pie tin; cover and refrigerate until you're ready for it.

Preheat the oven to 350°F. Whisk together all the remaining ingredients until they're well-mixed. Pour into pie shell and bake for 35 to 40 minutes, or until firm.

The Hemp Cookbook, Todd Dalotto

Hemp Brownies

8 tablespoons (1 stick) unsalted butter
1/8 cup unsweetened chocolate
1 1/2 cups sugar
2 large eggs
1 teaspoon pure vanilla extract
3/4 cup unbleached white flour
1/4 cup hemp protein flour
1/4 teaspoon salt
1/2 cup toasted hemp nuts

Preheat oven to 350°F. Line an 8-inch square pan with aluminum foil. Grease the foil and set the pan aside. In the microwave on a high setting, melt the butter and chocolate in a large bowl for 45 seconds, stir, and microwave for 45 seconds more. Stir until all chocolate is melted and the mixture is smooth.

Stir in the sugar, eggs, and vanilla extract until well blended. Stir in the white and hemp flours and salt until just blended. Stir in the hemp nuts, then spread the mixture into the prepared pan.

Bake for 30 to 35 minutes, until you can insert a toothpick in the center, and it comes out with chocolate crumbs on it. Do not over bake. Allow to cool on a wire rack. Use the edges of the foil as handles to lift the brownies out onto a cutting board. Remove the foil and cut brownies into squares.

Makes about 16 brownies.

The Galaxy Global Hemp Cookbook, Denis Cicero

Hempy Fruit Salad

1 cup watermelon chunks or balls
1 cup raspberries
1 cup blueberries
1 cup apple, chopped
1 mango
1 small honeydew melon
1 cantaloupe
2 cups strawberries, sliced
1/8 cup hemp seed oil
1/2 cup hemp nuts
1/4 cup mint leaves, finely chopped
1/4 cup fresh orange juice

Optional
1 teaspoon fresh ginger, grated
1/4 cup dried coconut
1 1/2 cups naturally sweetened vanilla yogurt (or soy yogurt)

Peel and seed the melons, apple and mango. Mix all fruit together in bowl.

Add the orange juice and any other optional items (ginger, coconut, etc.).

Add the hemp seed oil, hemp nuts and mint leaves, and allow for mixture to sit for about half an hour before serving.

Serves 6–8.

Hemp Butter: A Healthy Alternative

Hemp seeds truly are a versatile food. Hemp butter is very easy to make—all you need are hemp seeds and a grinder. Just about any kitchen appliance that grinds can work (obviously though, some work better than others—you'll just need to experiment). A food processor usually is adequate, especially if you process the seeds multiple times. Hand-cranked food grinders can work well, because the kernel is quite soft. Many report that a Champion juicer works best of all, producing a fine taste and smooth texture. The trick is to liberate as much oil as possible, thereby making it into a spread.

Hemp seed butter is extremely versatile. You can use it as a dip; it's a great addition to shakes, smoothies and sauces, can be used in desserts; or use it just as you would "normal" butter—to spread on bread, toast, crackers and the like.

To store hemp butter, keep it sealed and refrigerated to avoid having it turn rancid.

Hemp Milk

There are many recipes for hemp milk, all of which can vary slightly or substantially. This recipe can be modified to your taste. Try adding vanilla extract, cinnamon, nutmeg, pure maple syrup or chocolate syrup for variation.

3 cups water
1 cup hemp nuts
1–3 tablespoons honey or agave nectar

Blend all ingredients in a blender until smooth. Pour the milk through a sieve and chill. Serve cold or use in other cooking. Makes about 4 cups.

Hemp Nut Milk

1/2 cup hemp nuts and other raw nuts and seeds
1/2 cup water
1/2 cup apple juice

Grind 1/2 cup of hemp nut and other raw nuts and seeds (almonds and cashews also work great—be creative!) Add water, blend until smooth.

Add apple juice; liquefy. Add more water if desired.

Filter through a strainer if desired. (Personally, I like the unstrained texture.) Save the puree to spread on toast, add to soups, or whatever else you might like to try.

For chocolate hemp milk, mix in raw or roasted carob powder. *www.brendanbrazier.com*

About the Recipe Contributors

Todd DaLotto is the founder and owner of Hungry Bear Hemp Foods, the original producer of hemp seed snacks. He lives and cooks in the Coastal Range Mountains of Oregon.

Denis Cicero is the designer and owner of the Galaxy Global Eatery in New York City. He has been involved in the food industry for over twenty-three years, associated with more than thirty different restaurant concepts.

Chi Hemp Industries Incorporated (CHII) is headquartered in Victoria, British Columbia, Canada. This corporation is in the business of growing, supplying, facilitating and diversifying the commercial hemp industry, while encouraging a 100 percent sustainable approach to all aspects of the agriculture, industry and commerce associated with it.

Tonya Kay is a raw-food-athlete who has danced for over 2 years in the Off-Broadway phenomenon STOMP. Her cutting-edge choreography has been featured at Los Angeles's Sunset Room, New York City's Javits Center, and in theatre throughout Chicago. In addition she has taught tap and hip-hop at renowned studios all over the world.

Brendan Brazier is a professional vegan Ironman triathlete. He is the creator of Vega, the world's first hemp-based meal replacement. Brendan's full-length cookbook will be released in 2005. Visit his website at www.brendanbrazier.com.

References

Cicero, Denis. *The Galaxy Global Eatery Hemp Cookbook.* Frog Limited; Berkeley, California; 2002.

Conrad, Chris. *Hemp for Health: The Medicinal and Nutritional Uses of Cannabis Sativa.* Healing Art Press; Rochester, Vermont; 1997.

Dalotto, Todd. *The Hemp Cookbook.* Healing Arts Press; Rochester, Vermont; 2000.

Leson, Gero and Pless, Petra. Evaluating Interference in THC in Hemp Food Products with Employee Drug Testing. Leson Environmental Consulting, July 2000.

Robinson, Rowan, and Robert A. Nelson. *The Great Book of Hemp: The Complete Guide to the Commercial, Medicinal and Psychotropic Uses of the World's Most Extraordinary Plant.* Park Street Press; 1995.

Woodland Health Series

*Definitive Natural Health Information
At Your Fingertips!*

The Woodland Health Series offers a comprehensive array of single topic booklets, covering subjects from fibromyalgia to green tea to weight loss. If you enjoyed this title, look for other WHS titles at your local health-food store, or contact us. Complete and mail (or fax) us the coupon below and receive the complete Woodland catalog and order form—free!

Or . . .

- Call us toll-free at (800) 777-2665
- Visit our website
  (www.woodlandpublishing.com)
- Fax the coupon (and other correspondence) to
  (801) 334-1913

The Natural Choice for
Prostate Health

**Saw
Palmetto**

Immune and
Stamina Booster

**Cordyceps
Sinensis**

Kate
Gilbert
Udall

Potent Soy
Isoflavone

Genistein

Rita
Elkins,
M.H.
